Sex: When to Say "Yes"

A Bible Study for Young Adults on Sex
Fran & Jill Sciacca

World Wide Publications
Minneapolis, Minnesota 55403

Sex: When to Say "Yes"

World Wide Publications is the publishing division of the
Billy Graham Evangelistic Association.

ISBN: 0-89066-099-9

Printed in the United States of America

Why "Lifelines"?

Who in the world are Fran and Jill…is it Sky-Ocka??

The name "Sciacca" (actually pronounced "Shock-a") is probably not a familiar name to you. Let me take you on a quick trek through our lives, so you will know who we are and why we care so much about you.

Fran grew up in the shadow of older identical twin brothers who were football stars. While their photos and accomplishments appeared regularly in newspapers and magazines, Fran found himself wondering who he was besides "the twins' little brother." In high school, he decided to take his talents "elsewhere," completely out of the arena of athletics; he set out to become the best bass guitarist he could be. His rock band was a success, and soon Fran also made it to the pages of the newspaper. On one occasion he played in front of 5,000 people at a "battle of the bands" in Milwaukee, Wisconsin. Fame became Fran's total focus in his search for "self." He was popular at school and was elected class president for three years.

In college, Fran quickly blazed his way to the top of his fraternity. The professional status of his new rock group also gave him personal pride. The band's popularity soared beyond the college campus, and Fran began doing "warm-up" for nationally known entertainers such as Chase and B.J. Thomas. He had finally "arrived"–or so he thought. But why, he wondered, was the feeling of emptiness still lodged so deep in his soul?

Then in one year's time the band began to break up, his girlfriend dumped him, and he received the devastating news that one of his brothers had been seriously wounded in the Vietnam war. It was as if someone had let the air out of his world. He felt alone in the universe. Even his 12 years of religious education in a private school didn't help him.

About this time, God brought a friend into Fran's life who had just committed his own life to Jesus Christ. Late one night in a quiet dorm room, Fran heard from him about the depth of God's love. For the first time, Fran had reason to believe that he was a valuable person, not because he was "cool," or a popular bass guitarist but because the God of the universe loved him and had paid the penalty for his sin. Fran found the identity he had always longed for in the person of Jesus Christ.

Jill's Journey

I grew up in "the suburbs," graduating with a class of more than 700 students. My years in high school could best be characterized by my quest to know, "Where's the party?" But when I was alone, I often thought about life and death–even suicide. I wrote poems that exposed my inner fears, but felt they were "safe" as simple assignments for English class. As best I could, I squelched my spiritual emptiness by dancing, partying, working a little and playing a lot.

My folly and flippant approach to study in high school forced me to be on probation for the first quarter of college. I buckled down to get good grades, but somehow managed to maintain my carefree lifestyle "to the max." I was dating a gifted art student, and together with other friends we embraced the sixties counterculture. Our philosophy boasted that peace was possible; we could affect society and bring about lasting change. "We" were the answer to all of America's problems.

Yet in two years' time I witnessed the tragic folly of the sixties philosophy in vivid detail: a best friend from high school had burned out on drugs. Another had died while on drugs. I had seen that our protests against the Vietnam war were leading to prison sentences. People were losing heart. Dropping out. My boyfriend had been committed to a psychiatric ward in a hospital. My best girlfriend, who had entered college on a scholarship, had quit, disillusioned with life. My rock star heros had fallen from the thrones I'd placed them on. Jimi Hendrix had died. (I had been in the front rows at one of his concerts.) Jim Morrison was gone. Drugs and death seemed to go together. We were not the answer to America's woes–we were part of the problem!

So I fled from the fast lane and started studying philosophy, searching for answers but finding none. Finally, I desperately cried out to the God I had learned about in Sunday school as a child. I had always believed in him, but never realized that I could know him personally. Committing my life to him, I made him my Lord and found the peace I hadn't found in all my searching. I joined the ranks of the revival on our college campus, the one that had also swept Fran into the faith. We were radical, but now we had an anchor and a purpose that really was destined to succeed.

And Then, Fran & Jill

We were married after graduation from college. Our first home was in Wisconsin, out in the country, where we attended a small church. There we immediately gravitated to the youth. Three years and one son later, the Lord led us to Denver, Colorado, where Fran went to seminary. While in Denver, we were again drawn to teens as Fran did field work at a local church. Two years and another son later, the Lord led us to Colorado Springs Christian School, where Fran has been teaching high school Bible ever since! Now we also have the blessed bonus of twin daughters.

We needed to tell you all this for two reasons: First, everything that these studies deal with comes out of our own experience. Second, in many of the things that you're going to look at in *Lifelines: Getting a Hold on Life,* we totally "blew it." So not only do we understand the issues at hand, we also know the pain and temptation that go with the territory.

We believe that a genuine relationship with Jesus Christ and with those who are committed to him is the most fulfilling and exciting thing on this sometimes perplexing planet! We're not talking about people who "play church." We're talking about those who are really serious about falling in love with, and following, the One who died for us.

So be assured that your struggles are familiar to us. They are foes that we have fought too. They are battles that we often lost. But we know there is a way of victory, and we want to help you discover that door of hope.

We pray that, through a personal study of God's Word, you will gain a new vision for a meaningful life, walking with the Lord and living in victory.

Fran and I are a "fun" team. He is the "architect"; I am the "builder." You will find the Bible study section of each chapter designed by Fran. I have helped Fran put a "personal touch" to the studies by telling a story you can relate to, about someone who has been a part of our lives. (Names, gender and nonessential details have been altered to protect the privacy of those involved.)

There is one more thing we want you to know as you begin this Bible study–we really care about you!

What Is "Lifelines"?

Life is tough! Being a teenager is even tougher. You bounce somewhere between adulthood and childhood, ping-ponging back and forth, not really landing on either side, never really knowing which side you're supposed to be on at any given moment. The temptation to give in or give up may seem greater than you can bear. You probably feel as if you're sinking in a sea of pressures and problems too deep and wide to navigate. Let's face it, life's a battle. But…on the other hand, is that so unusual?

What does it take to make the first-string soccer team? What's the cost of working your way to first-chair trumpet in the school band? How long did you have to practice to become the best guitarist at school? Remember those early morning practices for the spring play? It seems as if everything significant has a price tag. Maybe that's the way it's supposed to be; maybe that's the way God planned it. But, he also provides the help we need along the way. *Lifelines: Getting a Hold on Life* is one of those helpers.

"Lifelines" Is Different.

Lifelines: Getting a Hold on Life is different. It won't help you "sail" through life, because nobody sails through life. But *Lifelines* will be honest with you about life, about God, about yourself, about your choices and your dreams. *Lifelines* promises to "put the cookies on the bottom shelf," to meet you right where you are and deal with the things that you have to deal with each day. It promises to provide answers where there are answers, and to ask questions where they need to be asked.

But, just as in the rest of life, there are some costs that go with these Bible studies. What are they? Simply this: *Lifelines: Getting a Hold on Life* promises to be honest with you, but you've got to be honest with yourself. And even more important–you've got to be honest with God. These studies are built on the presupposition that the Bible is God's Word. That means that your opinions and feelings have a genuine place in your life, but the final place is reserved for God's Word.

This Bible study cannot change your life; only God can do that. But, God can't guide a parked car. You're the one who's got to cooperate with God as you carefully work through this study.

You've got to be willing to let the Lord into your life, into your problems and pressures, into your battle. He wants to be beside you whether you are defeated or determined. If you are willing to pay this price, *Lifelines: Getting a Hold on Life* could very well be one of the most exciting things that happens to you this year!

Things to Keep in Mind:

Here are some important thoughts to keep in mind as you begin:

#1–God is not a coach. He doesn't have a checklist for your performance. He loves you. In fact, he loves you just as you are as you begin this study.

#2–Apply what you learn to yourself. Resist the urge to think of others who "really need to hear" what you are learning.

#3–Be faithful. Whatever your commitment is, whether to a group or simply to yourself, keep it. Make it your goal to finish the study.

#4–Be realistic. Weeds grow quickly, but an oak tree takes time. Look for small ways to grow. If you set goals that are too tough, you'll become discouraged. Small victories will encourage you to keep going.

Lifelines: Getting a Hold on Life accepts the fact that much of life is a battle for you. But, you can win.

> You've got to know there's a bigger plan.
> Room to fall, room to stand.
> Pray for the plan to begin in you.
> Keep your heart true.*
> [sung by Amy Grant]

God wants you to win the battle. But remember: *you can't have a victory where there's been no fight.* You may fall—we all do—but learn to stand!

How to Use This Bible Study

This Bible study is part of a series entitled *Lifelines: Getting a Hold on Life*. Each study in the series centers around a single issue that you as a teenager face in the twentieth century. This study, *Sex: When to Say "Yes,"* deals with the Bible's teaching regarding sex.

Each chapter of *Sex: When to Say "Yes,"* includes a real-life story, some personal study questions, and a summary discussion. Look for one major truth, a "Lifeline," as you go through each chapter. If there are specific things the study asks you to do, be sure to do them. The personal insights you pull out of these pages won't help you until you begin to put them into practice.

The only things you will need to complete this study are a Bible, a pen, and an open heart. We suggest that you use a version of the Bible that is easy to read, such as the New International Version or The Living Bible. Make sure that your Bible has both the Old and the New Testaments. We would suggest you also have a spiral notebook to record thoughts and ideas that come to you while you study.

If you study *Sex: When to Say "Yes"* in a group, you'll find the optional group discussion questions in each chapter's "Bottom Line" section enlightening and helpful.

There is another optional section near the end of each chapter entitled "His Lines." These are two passages from the Bible that might be helpful as you seek to make the "Lifeline" from that chapter a reality in your own life. You can memorize these verses, put them on your mirror, in your locker, or on the dashboard of your car. Plant them any place where they can prompt you to remember the truth when you need it the most.

Other Lifelines

If you enjoy studying *Sex: When to Say "Yes,"* you may want to try these other *Lifeline* studies:

Desperately Seeking Perfect Family Family

Burger, Fries and a Friend to Go Friendship

1

Is God a Cosmic Cop?

Opening Lines

Christmas is a challenging time of the year for my children. As we meander through the shopping malls, their little eyes become ablaze with selfish longing. Their appetites crave each new toy that television and friends have told them will satisfy all their wildest wishes. Their thoughts are not on giving gifts to others; rather, they are trapped in a revolving door, chasing their own desires. My children are convinced that life will be a tedious passing of time unless they possess a certain toy. Most frustrating for us as parents is the knowledge that these "needs" our children perceive they have are disastrous deceptions. They feel cheated because they've chosen to weep over what they don't have rather than being content and satisfied with the sufficient amount of toys they do have. At times this burning desire seems almost impossible to bear, both for them and for us!

I've run into a host of Christian high school students who feel just like my four children at Christmas. They covet and crave the freedom and liberty that the non-Christian flaunts before their eyes. Especially in the area of sex. High school girls have confessed to me that they go "cruisin" on weekends, searching for some good-looking "stud" to pick up. I recall one student in particular who blurted out in frustration, "The non-Christians have all the fun! They're the only ones who have good parties. Sometimes it seems as if God gets his kicks out of making me unhappy!"

This girl voiced the feeling of many Christian young people. Prime-time television displays a daily menu of sexual delights, most of which are outside of marriage. It deludes us into believing that sexual freedom is fulfilling and acceptable. The lyrics to much of the music we hear also advocate sexual freedom and experimentation. Clothing styles are often designed to excite and stimulate desire rather than flatter and draw attention to one's face. Sometimes living in America is like visiting a sexual carnival. The question for the Christian becomes: "Why shouldn't I go on these rides? Everyone else is!"

The Christian is confronted with confusing questions. What are God's standards in the area of sex? What are his motives? Is he some kind of cosmic cop, anxious to blow his whistle on anyone who starts to have fun?

On the Lines

1. What exactly does the Bible say about sexual intercourse outside of marriage? Look at the verses below and write out what God says about sex outside of marriage:

Ephesians 5:3 ____

____

1 Corinthians 6:18 ______________________________________

____

2. According to the two verses above, whom do you sin against when you have sex outside of marriage?

____

____

3. Even though God is clear about his attitude toward sex outside of marriage, it doesn't explain why he has set such a high standard or what he thinks of the various things that can lead up to sexual intercourse. Take the following "Facts and Fables Quiz" to examine your own understanding of the issues surrounding sex outside marriage:

FACTS AND FABLES QUIZ

Questions	*True*	*False*
Having permarital sex draws couples closer together.	☐	☐
Having premarital sex promotes a happier marriage.	☐	☐
Those who have premarital sex are less likely to become divorced later.	☐	☐
Premarital sex has very little effect on a person's ability to relate to God.	☐	☐
Those who have premarital sex are less likely to commit adultery when married.	☐	☐
Having premarital sex is a good way to help you know if the person is the right one to marry.	☐	☐
Those who have premarital sex have more satisfying sex lives while they are married.	☐	☐
Those who engage in premarital sex have fewer bad sex habits in marriage.	☐	☐

Look back over your answers. How many did you mark true? Wherever you marked true, you were wrong! Every one of the statements is false. This information is the result of professional studies done on hundreds and hundreds of relationships among people your age.

4. Now, let's look to see if the Bible can give us some clues concerning God's motive for such a high standard regarding sex outside of marriage. Look up the verses below and write down how God feels about you.

John 3:16 ____

John 14:21 ____

John 16:27 ____

1 John 4:9,10 ____

5. If God loves you, and premarital sex produces all the negative results seen in question 3, what must be his motive in forbidding premarital sex?

____

____

____

6. Summarize any new discoveries you have made about premarital sex from this chapter.

____

____

____

____

Between the Lines

1. Go back over the "Facts and Fables Quiz." Look at your answers.

Fill in the chart below. Put as many entries as you can under each heading. Be honest!

Benefits of premarital sex	*Penalties of premarital sex*
1.	1.
2.	2.
3.	3.
4.	4.
5.	5.
6.	6.
7.	7.
8.	8.
9.	9.

2. Now, write out what you believe about premarital sex as a result of this study.

My beliefs about premarital sex.

____

____

____

____

Closing Lines

God isn't a cosmic cop. He's your heavenly Father. He is a holy God, so breaking his commands is a sin against him. But, he is also a loving Father. It is his love for you in particular and his desire to protect you that motivates him to say "no" to premarital sex. Sex outside of marriage isn't just a sin against him; it's also a sin against yourself—you are the victim! The only benefit of premarital sex is the pleasure you receive while you do it. But the penalties are staggering! And because God loves you, he wants to protect you from those penalties.

Even though you live in an age in which sex is promoted as America's number one sport, God's standard is that it is a forbidden fruit outside of marriage. But, his motive is his love for you—a love that cost him his Son's life!

Lifeline:

God says "no" to premarital sex because he loves me.

His Lines

1 Corinthians 6:18

Hebrews 13:4

The Bottom Line (For Group Discussion)

1. If most Americans get married more than once, why should you be a virgin for your first marriage?

2. Discuss answers to question 1 of "Between the Lines."

3. What do you think are the greatest sources of sexual temptation? Why?

2

The Law of Locust Years

Opening Lines

Michelle was a broken girl. Over a period of three years she had progressively become more physically involved with her boyfriend. Having sex had become a regular part of their relationship. An unwanted pregnancy, however, surprised them both and ended in an agreed-upon abortion. Then, with almost as little advance warning as the pregnancy, Michelle's boyfriend dumped her. Three years of her life slipped out of her grasp in a single evening! She was abruptly alone.

In an attempt to rebuild her ruined life, Michelle started to get serious with God. She concluded that a genuine relationship with Jesus Christ was the only hope for her. But her feelings of guilt were overwhelming. The pain of her lost virginity, a concealed and cancelled pregnancy, and a shattered love affair lingered in her memory like a living nightmare. "Can Christ really forgive me?" she constantly questioned. "Can he put the pieces of my life back together without too many cracks for the world to see?"

Just what can God do for those whose lives have been scarred by sexual sin? Is he as good as the detergents on TV? Can God get the stains out?

On the Lines

1. The first concern that Michelle wanted to deal with was the crushing weight of guilt she carried. Look up the following verses and write out what you discover about God's forgiveness:

Ephesians 1:7 ________________________________

____

1 John 1:9 __________________________________

____

2. God promises to forgive. But aren't there some sins that God is less willing to forgive? Look at Michelle's sad story of premarital sex and abortion; do you think God wants to forgive such serious sins? Even if Michelle knew she was wrong all along? Look up the verses below and record God's answers to these questions:

Micah 7:18 __________________________________

____

Isaiah 1:18 __________________________________

____

3. God also makes a precious promise to anyone who turns to Jesus Christ as Savior, who takes that initial step to become a Christian. What is that promise?

2 Corinthians 5:17 ____________________________

____

How do you think this applies to someone who has lost his or her virginity?

____

____

____

4. Forgiveness from sin and guilt is an awesome thing. But, what about the consequences of sexual sin, the emotional pain and memories that somehow seem to linger? Can God give back what was lost here too? Can God really rebuild a person's life such as Michelle's? Look at the promises below and write out how you think they apply to someone's life that has been "eaten up" by sexual sin:

Joel 2:25 ____

____

____

Isaiah 61:7 ____

____

____

Zechariah 9:11,12 ____

____

____

5. Look at John 8:1–11. In this story, Jesus states the one requirement that he demands in order for our burdens to be lifted. What is that requirement (vs. 11)?

____

____

What do you think this involves? ________________________

____

____

6. Summarize what you've discovered about God's desire for you regarding failure in the area of sexual sin.

____

____

____

____

Between the Lines

1. God wants to "repay you for the years the locusts have eaten." But, sometimes that means getting rid of, or away from, the "locusts"! Under the heading "Locusts," write out the names of people or places that are a source of sexual sin or temptation for you. Then under the heading "Locust Killers," write out what you need to do to get out of that situation or environment. (*Hint:* This could be painful for you, but it is a necessity if you really want to regain lost ground in the area of sexual purity.)

LOCUSTS	LOCUST KILLERS

2. Talk to your best friend (same sex) about your decisions to drive out the "locusts." You don't have to mention any of the names. Ask this friend to help you to be faithful to your commitment for one month.

Closing Lines

Sexual sin pillages our lives like a plague of locusts. It can devastate our spiritual life, self-esteem, emotional health, and even our good friendships. It may provide immediate pleasure and feelings of acceptance, but then it demands to be "paid back" for a lifetime!

But Jesus Christ offers the opportunity for a person to regain his or her purity in *his* eyes when he or she becomes a Christian. He also promises forgiveness and restored fellowship to the Christian who sins but then truly repents. He offers to lift the load of guilt and "repay you for the years the locusts have eaten." God can and will rebuild the lives of those who genuinely desire to be pure in his eyes. But, he cannot do it unless you are serious about letting him! And that means you must flee from the "locusts" in your life—those people and places or things that lead or tempt you into sexual sin. Also, you must give God time. It isn't fair for you to demand or expect instant healing. I tell my students to give God at least as much time to put their life back together as they spent taking it apart.

Michelle is a fun-loving, fulfilled person today. No, the memories of her high school days aren't totally gone. But now they serve to remind her of God's marvelous love and ability to rebuild, rather than reminding her of her own guilt and shame. Michelle is a whole person today because of God's desire and adequacy to "repay you for the years the locusts have eaten." But Michelle is also healed because she willingly submitted to taking some painful yet necessary steps to cooperate with God in the process.

Lifeline:

God can restore the years the locusts have eaten.

His Lines

Joel 2:25

Matthew 11:28–30

The Bottom Line (For Group Discussion)

1. Why is it so painful to regain lost ground in the area of sex?

2. What are some ways to avoid sexual temptation and sin?

3. In what activities can your group participate to help one another stay away from sexually oriented situations?

4. What should be your involvement with sexually oriented television, movies, and magazines? Why?

5. What role does the way we dress play in sexual sin and temptation? What clothing styles do guys wear that are most sexually stimulating for girls? And what girls' fashions are most stimulating for guys? What responsibility do we have toward one another as Christians in the way we dress? Explain.

3

Supply and Demand

Opening Lines

It was insane! Sliding down the side of a small mountain at breakneck speed on snow that glistened like polished glass would have been excitement enough. But we were taking the trip on inner tubes!

About twenty of us had decided to go tubing one terribly cold mid-December Saturday morning. In a nearby town there was a recreational area that was identical to a downhill ski operation, except that you rented inner tubes instead of skis.

At first, everyone was admittedly scared. It takes courage to slide at lightning-like speed down a steep, slick slope in something you can't steer! But following a few safe runs, the whole group was loosening up, laughing and having a terrific time. Then slowly our fears were repressed and replaced with a suicidal daring on each new run. Before long we were spreading out five or six tubes and linking ourselves together like human chains as we whipped wildly down the hill. Some were layering themselves on top of each other like sandwiches, screaming down the slope like a human apartment building! Others were attempting to conquer the downhill quest standing up! We even grabbed one poor guy and piled six tubes over his head like donuts, smacked him on his side, and sent him soloing out of control down the hill. It took him awhile to recover from that one!

By the end of the day we had experimented with every conceivable combination of human beings and inner tubes. One daring guy who dove in front of two tied-together tubes descending the mountain had seriously dislocated his knee, but the rest of us reached the end of the day still standing. What is it in us that progressively produces dissatisfaction with one level of excitement and drives us on to something more? Why is it that what seems fun at the beginning of an adventure slowly wears out and we find ourselves looking for something more pleasurable, more exciting, and more satisfying? Why is it that holding hands on a date is enjoyable and fun at first, but we soon find ourselves wanting to make out or even go further? Is there some magical rule that controls all this?

On the Lines

1. James 1:13–15 provides a great deal of insight into this issue. According to this verse, what is the progression that occurs?

_______________leads to _________________________________

which leads to ____

2. The story of two of King David's children, Amnon and Tamar, vividly illustrates what James is talking about. Look at 2 Samuel 13:1–19. What verses in this story deal with Amnon's desire?

____

What verses in this story deal with Amnon's sin?

____

What verses in this story deal with "death" in Amnon's life?

____

---

3. Did Amnon's involvement with Tamar satisfy his desires? __

Explain ____

____

4. Proverbs 5 is a chapter that speaks clearly about the dangers of sex outside of marriage (specifically, adultery). Look at verses 18– 20. Where does God say he intends you to find sexual fulfillment?

---

5. In God's plan, sexual fulfillment is to be found within marriage. It also seems to be a part of his plan that sexual behavior is designed to lead up to sexual intercourse. In other words, God has planned it that certain sexual behavior cannot satisfy, because it is intended to lead to something more. And that something more is sexual intercourse, which God has reserved for marriage. This means that those who are not married have to guard their sexual behavior so they don't find themselves in situations where they are "over the edge," so to speak, with their sexual desires.

The "cliff of desire" on the next page illustrates our sexual behavior. The top of the cliff represents being together and the bottom of the valley represents sexual intercourse. This is what I want you to do:

Fill in on the illustration where you would put the following activities:

- holding hands
- goodnight kiss
- long kiss
- making out
- petting
- heavy petting

NOTE: As you fill in the illustration, put the one behavior that would cause you to begin thinking about sexual intercourse at the edge of the cliff. Be honest!

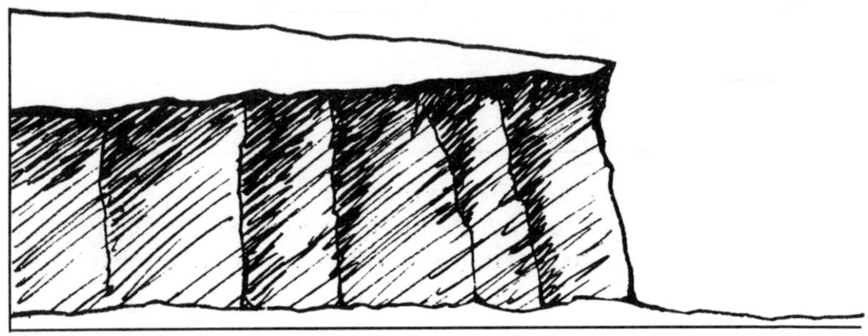

6. The one behavior you put on the edge is your "Point of No Return." This is the conduct that will lead you ultimately to engage in sexual intercourse. Which one of the following questions do you think you should ask yourself?

☐ How far away from this point must I be to be safe?

☐ How close to this point can I get before I'm in danger?

7. Explain your answer to question 6. __________

____

____

8. Does your life agree with your answers to questions 6 and 7? Explain.

____

____

____

9. Summarize any new discoveries about sex you have made as a result of this chapter.

Between the Lines

1. Write out your views on kissing, petting, and intercourse.

____

____

____

____

____

____

____

____

2. Would you be willing to give your love life to Jesus? Write him a letter to that effect and keep it someplace where you will see it often, but others won't.

3. If you have a good relationship with your parents, sit down with them some evening and ask what their views are on kissing, petting, and intercourse.

Closing Lines

By God's design, sexual demand always exceeds supply, unless it is within the freedom of marriage. There exists a "law of diminishing returns" for sexual behavior outside of marriage. If you engage in sexual behavior before marriage, the excitement and pleasure it provides at first will eventually dwindle and even disappear. The pleasure will return only if you move further toward the edge of your "cliff of desire" and eventually go over the edge. This law of diminishing returns is like the law of gravity; it works whether you believe it or not!

One question still remains—"Why did God give such strong sexual desires before you can legitimately fulfill them?" That question plagues almost every high-school-age person. I have asked it repeatedly myself, but I have come to realize that for you it really wouldn't make any difference if I could provide a perfectly logical and sound answer. The real issue is that sexual involvement is fun, and is pleasurable, and people do enjoy it. The bottom line is not really your need to know why, as much as that something inside you wants to acknowledge it's all right.

So, the real issue is not *why,* but *what.* What will your standards be? What choices will you make? What decisions will you make to guard your future? And today is the day these questions need to be answered.

Lifeline:

In sex outside of marriage, demand is always greater than supply.

His Lines

2 Samuel 13:14,15

Psalm 119:9

The Bottom Line (For Group Discussion)

1. What effect do sexually explicit TV, music, and movies have on our sex drive?

2. What are reasonable safeguards to prevent premarital sex?

3. What should you do if you can't seem to say "no" to the sexual temptations you face?

4. Who has more pressure to give in to sexual sin, guys or girls? Explain your answer.

5. Is masturbation a valid way to deal with sexual temptation? Explain your answer.

4

The Law of Stolen Water

Opening Lines

I was nervous. The clerk had been noticing me more frequently the past few minutes. I had been piling up magazines from the rack as I pretended to be seriously browsing. My stack totaled about six by now, and I was casually glancing at the saleslady who was serving the customers seated at the counter. I was a popular patron at our local drugstore, so my presence didn't normally create suspicion. But today, for some reason, the lady seemed to sense that I was up to something. Then, my big break beckoned. A man called for a cup of coffee, and she had to turn her back to me to help him. I hustled out the door and I was history! My heart hammered inside me as I accelerated my pace all the way home. I ran the mile sprint in record time. After I got inside, I waited for at least thirty minutes, fully expecting the phone to ring. I was confident that the clerk would report the theft to my parents. But, the call never came. Relieved, I put my feet up and began to enjoy the car magazines I had just stolen. I felt a sense of conquest, knowing that I was savoring something I hadn't paid for.

This feeling reached an alarming peak one day when I stole six yo-yos at the same time! I didn't need any yo-yos, let alone six! It began to dawn on me that I was now stealing just for the sake of stealing. I was taking things I didn't need or want just to provide me with the thrill of getting something illegitimately. The thought of going into a store and paying cash for something seemed totally boring and senseless. I had lost the ability to enjoy things in their proper setting. Something had robbed me of the rightful joy of ownership that comes from things legitimately acquired. What was it?

On the Lines

1. Look at Proverbs 9:17. What do you think it means that stolen water is "sweet"?

____

____

____

2. Why do you think this is the case? __________________________

____

____

3. Do you see any connection with my own feelings in the concluding section of "Opening Lines" and your answers to questions 1 and 2?

____

____

____

4. If you were to apply the principle from Proverbs 9:17 to premarital sex, what would the "stolen water" be?

____

5. Why would it be stolen? _______________________

____

____

6. Why would it be sweet? _______________________

____

____

7. If you take this "law of stolen water" from Proverbs 9:17, and combine it with what happened to me in the concluding section of "Opening Lines," what do you think could happen to those who had engaged in premarital sex when they get married and can have legitimate sex?

____

____

____

____

8. How would you answer the following questions?

Question	True	False
(1) Women who have sex before marriage are less likely to fully enjoy sex in marriage.	☐	☐
(2) Women who have sex before marriage are often bitter and hostile to their husbands after they are married.	☐	☐

(3) Husbands who have had sex with their wife
     before marriage feel she is less sexually respon-
     sive after they are married.   ☐   ☐

(4) Being sexually experienced before marriage
     does not improve sexual adjustment and fulfill-
     ment in marriage.   ☐   ☐

9. If you answered "false" to any of the above questions, you are
mistaken on that point. The answers are all true. How do you think
what you've discovered about the "law of stolen water" could
explain statements 1 and 3 in question 8? ___________________

____

____

____

10. Summarize any new discoveries you have made about the
subject of sex and the Christian from this chapter. ___________

____

____

____

Between the Lines

1. Perhaps you are already quite experienced in the area of sex. It
is not too late to set a new personal goal for your life. You can
begin today!

☐ Take some time before you go to sleep tonight and tell
   God what you've come to realize about your behavior. Tell
   him you are sorry and ask his forgiveness. (I would suggest
   that you do this kneeling.) If there are individuals you have
   sinned against sexually, I would suggest that you ask their

forgiveness as well. (Do it in person or over the phone. Do not do it in written form!)

☐ Make a short list of the steps you need to take to insure that you really will stop "stealing water." (This could be people you will quit hanging around with, places you will quit going to, or people you will start hanging around with and places you will start going to.)

☐ Check off the items on your list as you do them.

2. If you know of someone older of the same sex that you can confide in, do it. Tell him or her of your struggles and your new goals. Ask that person to pray for you and to ask once a week how it's going for two months.

Closing Lines

One of the key requirements for getting a good job is experience. Employers are looking for people who know what to do. In God's design for sex, the opposite is true. He's looking for people who aren't experienced, people who haven't got a lot of sexual skills.

God's intention is that one man and one woman will learn together over a lifetime. In the process of becoming experienced, a beautiful thing happens—they become "one." But if we engage in premarital sex, we not only thwart God's plan, but we also develop a taste for a pleasure in sex that is often missing when we actually get married. The Lord calls this the "law of stolen water." Illegitimate sex provides a certain thrill that is not the result of sex itself, but rather is the consequence of stealing pleasures that don't belong to us.

Statistics show that those who engage in premarital sex are much more likely to be unfaithful and unfulfilled in marriage. The "law of stolen water" means that sex is *rightfully owned* in marriage and does not satisfy the desire one has developed from stealing it, in the form of premarital sex. The natural response to this is for that marriage partner to go looking for such pleasure outside of marriage. This is a crucial concept for you to grasp right now, because statistics state that nine out of ten of you will get married (even if you say, "Not me! I'll *never* get married!").

According to God's Word, "stolen water is sweet." I cannot deny that. But, there's another verse in the Bible that talks about the "law of stolen water" that you need to be aware of too:

> Food gained by fraud tastes sweet to a man,
> But he ends up with a mouth full of gravel.
>
> [Proverbs 20:17]

Lifeline:

Sex before marriage can ruin sex in marriage.

His Lines

Proverbs 5:20,21

Proverbs 20:17

The Bottom Line (For Group Discussion)

1. Why do you think the world puts such an emphasis on having sexual experience?

2. Why do you think God doesn't?

3. Have your group do a survey of students at their schools, using the questions from question 8 in "On the Lines." Discuss the answers they received. (NOTE: Keep track of male vs. female answers.)

5

Missionary Dating?

Opening Lines

"But, you don't know Bruce, Mr. Sciacca," Joy argued, her eyes begging me to change my mind. "He's different. In fact, he has higher standards than the Christian guys I've dated!" Her last comment caused me great physical and emotional distress. It disgusted me. I had heard it too many times before to dismiss it.

Sitting in my office was an attractive, intelligent Christian girl. A typical sophomore in high school, she was seeking a wholesome relationship with a guy who would respect and honor her for who she was. Someone to be seen with and someone to have fun with. So, she accepted a few dates from "outstanding young Christian men," only to discover that they couldn't keep their hands off her and didn't have a clue as to how to treat a young woman with respect or care.

With this bitter experience of a few bad "Christian" dates fresh in her memory, Bruce steps on the scene. He's bright, funny, honest, and has high moral standards. His conduct on their first date left Joy's head and heart happily spinning. They had enjoyed a marvelous time together, talking and laughing, and as the night came to a close, he walked her to the door, kissed her lightly on her forehead, and said, "Thanks for a wonderful time, Joy. Can I call you again?" "Can you call me again?! Can you call me again?!"

she mused. Trying to contain her excitement, she had casually responded, "Sure. I would like that." As he drove away, she stared out the window and reminisced about the evening. She hadn't had to say, "Please, don't." He had actually looked at her when he talked or she talked, he had opened doors for her, and he had asked her about her church involvement with genuine interest. He told her he admired her religious beliefs, and that he was glad she had found something to believe in. Bruce wasn't a Christian—yet. But Joy felt sure she could change all that (with God's help of course!).

So there I sat, delicately trying to sort through Joy's "no win" choices. She could date the Christian guys she knew and be grossed out by their behavior, or she could date a non-Christian like Bruce who really treated her with respect, or she could sit home and sulk on weekends. It certainly did seem unfair. Maybe she could lead Bruce to the Lord. Maybe this was God's will for her life. Or was it?

On the Lines

1. Look up the word "yoke" in the dictionary and write the definition below.

____

____

2. Now, look at 2 Corinthians 6:14,15. Using your answer from question 1 to help you understand this passage, do you think Paul is speaking only of marriage, or of relationships with non-Christians in general?

____

Explain. ______________________________________

____

____

3. God forbids marriage to nonbelievers for Christians. But, what about dating a non-Christian? The Bible is silent on the subject specifically, but God has provided us with many principles about life in general that we can weave together to get an answer to our question.

(a) The starting point for the Christian, for every area of life is found in Matthew 22:34–38. Write out Jesus' answer in your own words:

____

____

____

(b) Our values are the things that we believe are the most important issues in life. 1 John 2:15–17 gives a brief comparison between the value system of a Christian and the value system of a non-Christian. Think hard, then describe what you see as the value system of each from this passage:

Non-Christian's value system

____

____

____

____

Christian's value system

____

____

____

____

(c) Jesus gives a sobering picture of two groups of people in Matthew 7:24–27. One group represents the obedient Christian and the other the disobedient Christian. The picture Jesus paints has to do with the very foundation of a person's life, that on which everything else depends. What does Jesus say here?

____

____

____

____

4. Now let's go back over the study you've done so far and piece together some critical principles that will cast some light on the question of dating non-Christians.

(a) Do you think it is possible for a Christian to fall in love with a non-Christian? ☐ Yes ☐ No

(b) If it did happen, what choices would the Christian be forced to make? (use your answer to question 3a)

____

____

____

(c) Be honest here. If the Christian chose God, do you think it would be a painful choice? Explain your answer.

____

____

____

5. Let's assume our Christian in question 4 did not choose God, but instead chose the boyfriend or girlfriend. Looking at your answers to question 3b and 3c, describe what you guess would happen if they were to marry.

____

____

____

____

____

____

6. Summarize any new discoveries you have made from this chapter about dating non-Christians.

____

____

____

Between the Lines

1. Are you in a "missionary dating" situation? Is it working? If not, what steps do you believe you need to take as a result of what you've learned from this chapter?

2. Are you willing to stay home on date nights, if it becomes necessary, in order to preserve your "priority love affair" with Jesus?

3. Find a friend who is struggling with the same issue and spend time together in prayer for strength and courage.

Closing Lines

God does not say "no" to a Christian who wants to date a nonbeliever (although he does oppose their getting married). In fact, the real issue is not the date itself, but rather the possible consequence. It is very possible for a Christian to fall in love with a nonbeliever. I have seen it happen too often to think otherwise. Relationships with the opposite sex often cause our consciences and convictions to take a back seat to our emotions. Our feelings become our guides, and those feelings are not the best guardians for our souls.

If you fall in love with a non-Christian, you will be tempted to try to live somewhere between being a Christian and a non-Christian. I need to be honest with you—this "somewhere between" zone doesn't exist! The real issue is that you will be forced to choose between Jesus Christ and your boyfriend or girlfriend. If Jesus loses, you will be building your house upon the sand, and it will eventually collapse.

But what about continuing the relationship so that you can win him or her to the Lord? You may even see yourself as the only Christian influence in his or her life! Let me pass on to you what I did with Joy that day. I had her stand on the desk in my room (we were the only ones in there!) and grab my hand. Then I said, "Joy, I want you to pull me up onto the desk." She grunted and groaned as she yanked on my arm. The best she could do was to get me up on my tiptoes momentarily. Then I looked at her soberly and said, "Hang on!" With one sharp pull, I jerked her off the desk and onto the floor. Looking down, I swiftly said, "Do you get the point?" She did. She knew that trying to pull Bruce up to Christ was less realistic than his pulling her down. Joy ended her "missionary dating" with Bruce. In time, he went totally "down the tubes" in terms of drugs and drinking. But do you know something? Joy would have eventually been there with Bruce. Oh, she could have possibly postponed him from doing what he did for a while, but it would have been only temporary. I know; I've seen too many students who didn't have the courage and conviction that led Joy to leave Bruce.

So, dating non-Christians isn't forbidden, but it's potentially hazardous to your spiritual health. Dangerous. If you decide that you still want to date a non-Christian, I ask that you be totally faithful to these four steps:

#1—Have your standards established before you start the relationship. What are your sexual limits? What places will you not go? What will you do if your date does not respect your standards? You must have answers to all of these questions before you begin the relationship.

#2—Establish that you are a Christian early in the relationship. I suggest that you make this clear before your first time together. The longer you wait to establish that Jesus is your "first love," the harder it will be to do so later on.

#3—Maintain your personal relationship with Jesus. It is imperative that you spend time in prayer and in the Bible on a regular basis.

#4—You must be willing to break off the relationship if you cannot maintain the first three of these steps. This is a decision that you must have already made at the beginning of the relationship, not in the middle of it.

Dating is a risky business in itself, and dating a non-Christian complicates it even more. Having thought through the issues beforehand and having defined limits and choices before you go into a relationship are the best assurances that it will be positive and beneficial rather than destructive and harmful.

Lifeline:

Missionary dating can be hazardous to your spiritual health.

His Lines

2 Corinthians 6:14,15

Matthew 22:34–38

The Bottom Line (For Group Discussion)

1. Why do you think Christians sometimes have lower moral standards than non-Christians?

2. Is having a date on the weekends important to you? Explain.

3. It is common for a couple to believe that their spiritual life is not a vital issue in marriage. Why do you think they feel this way?

4. Is it enough that the person you marry can say honestly that he or she is a Christian, or do you believe there needs to be a high level of commitment in his or her Christian life? Explain.

6

Different!
Opening Lines

Carmen was crushed. It was obvious from the tears tumbling down her face and the pain in her voice as she poured out her problem to me. "He made me feel like the most special person in the whole world," she sighed. "He called, he listened, he helped me through some tough times with my parents. He was such a good friend." Then she really started to sob, "But all of a sudden he quit calling, and when I tried to confront him at school, he treated me like dirt!" Carmen's crisis was not only a common one I had faced in counseling high school students, it was the third time I had heard the identical story about the same guy!

Bill was a "womanizer," one of those winsome guys who travels from girl to girl, leaving a trail of broken hearts behind him like eggshells at an omelet parlor! The story was always the same: He would initiate a casual interest in a girl during class, talk to her more and more frequently for the next few weeks, and finally ask her out. Then Bill would call every evening encouraging the girl to open up to him. It seemed that just about the time he succeeded in getting the girl really to reveal her heart to him, sharing her deepest secrets, he would dump her and begin the process all over again with someone new.

Observing Bill's "hit and run" behavior with so many of my

baffled and bitter female students, I kept asking myself, "Doesn't this guy see what he's doing to these girls?" I was also puzzled by the fact that Bill could date and dump one girl and then start the process over again with her best friend—and he was able to pull it off! But, the truth eventually became clear to me; neither Bill nor his female classmates were really aware of the differences between guys and girls. Consequently they didn't have a clue how to treat one another correctly. How should guys and girls act toward one another? Are there really significant differences between them? If so, what are they?

On the Lines

1. One of the key differences between guys and girls has to do with how they are stimulated sexually. Understanding this basic truth can help you to know how to act around members of the opposite sex. Look at Matthew 5:27, 28 and 2 Samuel 11:2 and 4. Using these two passages as a basis, how does it appear that men are stimulated sexually?

____

____

2. Should this have any influence on how a Christian girl dresses?

____

Explain. ____

____

____

3. Although men are stimulated sexually by sight, women are stimulated by touch. What effect should this truth have on the way guys behave around girls, even on a casual basis?

____

---

4. Probably the single greatest difference between guys and girls is in the way each of them perceives and projects love. Men tend to view love as physical and visible, with an emphasis on the present. Women, on the other hand, tend to view love as romantic and mental, and frequently project the relationship into the future.

Using these differences as your information, take the "Differences Quiz" below. Select only one answer for each statement. Check your answers on page 51.

DIFFERENCES QUIZ

Statement	*Guys*	*Girls*
(a) Would tend to recall only the pleasure associated with a goodnight kiss.	☐	☐
(b) Would tend to consider being asked out on a date a possible indication that the person had a romantic interest in him or her.	☐	☐
(c) Would tend to look for character qualities more than appearance as the reason to want to date someone.	☐	☐
(d) Would tend to consider sharing inner secrets with someone as evidence of a deep and lasting relationship.	☐	☐
(e) Would tend to use physical attractiveness as the primary determining factor in asking someone out.	☐	☐
(f) Would tend to view notes, phone calls and special gifts as evidence of a deep and lasting relationship.	☐	☐
(g) Would tend to view physical involvement as an expression of commitment.	☐	☐
(h) Would tend to view sharing inner secrets as just an interesting activity.	☐	☐
(i) Would tend to consider a date an experiment to determine what a person is like.	☐	☐

(j) Would tend to view flirting as a game.   ☐   ☐

(k) Would tend to think about "what might be" in a
     dating relationship.   ☐   ☐

(l) Would view flirting as an indicator that the per-
     son was sexually available.   ☐   ☐

5. Look back over the correct answers to the "Differences Quiz".
Can you pinpoint any attitudes or behavior on your part that could
be misleading to your date, or even to friends of the opposite sex?

What are they? ____

____

____

____

6. Look at Romans 14:13. How does it relate to your answer in
question 5?

____

____

7. Summarize any new discoveries you have made about how to
act or not to act around members of the opposite sex.

____

____

____

Between the Lines

1. Look over your answers to question 5 of "On the Lines." Pick one thing and make a commitment to work on that one area this entire week.

2. What are you communicating by the way you dress?

3. Is there a relationship in your life in which you are misleading the person? Take some time this week to be open and honest with that person about what you really want for your relationship.

Closing Lines

The differences between men and women are distinct and significant. Bill's involvement with Carmen (and other girls) was very misleading. The special interest communicated to her and the considerate attention he gave were interpreted by Carmen to be evidences of a romantic interest on his part. Her way of convincing him that she also felt attracted to him was in the form of privileged information, her personal private thoughts. But in many cases, what is surrendered by the girl is ownership to her body—sexual involvement. For girls this is a costly surrender, but one they are willing to pay in order to prove to a guy that they are attracted to him and would like the relationship to continue into the future.

Unfortunately, most guys are just like Bill and cannot see or plan beyond the present. Their sexual involvement with a girl is never looked upon as an investment or a risk on their part. It is merely an activity, an activity to be enjoyed in the present. So, a guy interprets sexual liberty given by a girl to mean that she enjoys it as much as he does, nothing more! The girl's message of coveted commitment never gets communicated to the guy.

Realizing how a girl perceives and projects love, guys, especially Christian guys, need to be very careful that they are not misleading the girls they date or hang around with.

Also, because guys are so quickly stimulated visually, I believe a Christian girl has a real responsibility to be modest and discreet in the way she dresses. A good rule of thumb is: Whatever you want a guy to love you for is what you should use to attract him. If a girl longs for a guy to love her for who she is, then she shouldn't use her careless outward appearance to attract him! I have counseled far too many girls who are convinced that the only thing their boyfriend loves them for is their body, yet that is precisely the "advertising" they used to attract him in the first place!

Dating should be a fun and maturing experience. You will make some mistakes for sure, but you can minimize the possible damages if you'll take to heart some of the principles covered in this chapter. Remember, people are treasures, not opportunities.

Lifeline:

Guys and girls interpret relationships totally differently.

His Lines

Proverbs 27:5

Proverbs 29:5

The Bottom Line (For Group Discussion)

1. One researcher compiled a list of the lines guys use on girls to get them sexually stimulated and involved. Here are a few of them. From what you've learned in this study, discuss why guys would use them, and why girls would respond.

> "Don't worry, you won't get pregnant."

> "If you get pregnant, I'll marry you."

> "I love you."

> "It's late. Why don't you stay overnight—I promise you I won't touch you."

> "I can't stop now."

> "Everybody's doing it."

> "Let's go upstairs."

> "Let's listen to records."

> "You have beautiful eyes."**

**Taken from *Youthletter*, page 93, 1977. Copyright Evangelical Ministries, Inc.

2. How do special dating events such as proms and homecoming tend to "punish" those who don't have dates?

3. Do you think group dating is more safe and fair than solo dating? Explain. (Note: This would be a good issue to debate in your group. Be sure to establish ground rules that would prohibit anyone getting hurt. Perhaps it would be best to assign those who are popular daters to defend the "group date" side of the debate.)

ANSWERS TO DIFFERENCES QUIZ

a.	guys		g.	girls
b.	girls		h.	guys
c.	girls		i.	guys
d.	girls		j.	girls
e.	guys		k.	girls
f.	girls		l.	guys